CHRISTOPHER ZANDERHOLM

One-Hour Workouts for the Athlete in their 40's, 50's, and 60's.

Making your body type work for you.

To my mother Sandra, who visited me everyday for six months while I was in the hospital.
Look how far I have come...

To Dr. Trevor Bachmeyer, for giving me my mindset reset. Never Miss.

To Kat V, for getting my ass back in the gym.

"The resistance that you fight physically in the gym and the resistance that you fight in life can only build a strong character."

-Arnold Schwarzenegger

Contents

1

Introduction and Overview

Welcome to "One-Hour Workouts for Athletes in their 40's, 50's, and 60's." It is a transformational journey that defies the odds and redefines what it means to prioritize health and fitness at any age. My name is Christopher Zanderholm, I stand before you not just as a guide, but as living proof that with determination, resilience, and the right tools, even the most daunting health challenges can be overcome.

My journey to health and wellness was far from conventional. In 2008, a seemingly routine medical procedure spiraled into a nightmare of infections, surgeries, and prolonged hospital stays. From battling a life-threatening infection that ravaged my hip and pelvis to enduring years of debilitating pain and physical limitations, I faced obstacles that would have shattered the resolve of many.

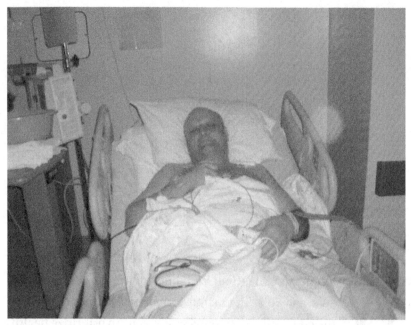

In recovery after a nine hour reconstructive surgery of my femur, hip, and pelvis.

But through it all, one thing remained steadfast: my unwavering commitment to reclaiming my health and rebuilding my life. It was a journey fraught with setbacks, moments of despair, and seemingly insurmountable obstacles. Yet, with each setback, I found the strength to rise again, fueled by a relentless determination to defy the odds and emerge stronger than before.

It is from this place of profound personal experience that "One-Hour Workouts for Athletes in their 40's, 50's, and 60's." was born. This book is not just a collection of exercises and routines; it is a testament to the power of perseverance and the transformative potential of embracing an active lifestyle. Through its pages, I share the insights, strategies, and workouts that helped me not only regain my physical strength but also rediscover my zest for life.

The Philosophy Behind the Approach

In a world that often correlates aging with decline, this book stands as a beacon of empowerment. The guiding principle is simple yet profound: age should enrich, not restrict, our fitness journey. We're challenging the narrative that suggests our best years are behind us, proposing instead that they can be right now with the right approach, mindset, and tools at our disposal. It's for the athlete who understands the value of time and seeks efficiency without compromise on quality.

When I use the word "athlete," I do so with the understanding that each and every one of us is an athlete in our own right. From the beginner athlete taking their first steps into the world of exercise to the seasoned athlete honing their craft, this book is for anyone who seeks to unleash their potential and take their life back into their own hands.

Whether you're juggling the demands of work, family, and personal life or facing health challenges that seem insurmountable, know this: "One-Hour Workouts for Athletes in their 40's, 50's, and 60's" is here to guide you every step of the way. With workouts designed to fit seamlessly into your busy schedule and strategies to overcome any obstacle that stands in your path, this book is your road map to success.

So, if you're ready to reclaim your health, reignite your passion for life, and unleash the athlete within, join me on this journey. Together, we will defy the odds, shatter limitations, and embrace a life of boundless possibility. Welcome to a new chapter in your story. Welcome to "One-

Hour Workouts for Athletes in their 40's, 50's, and 60's."

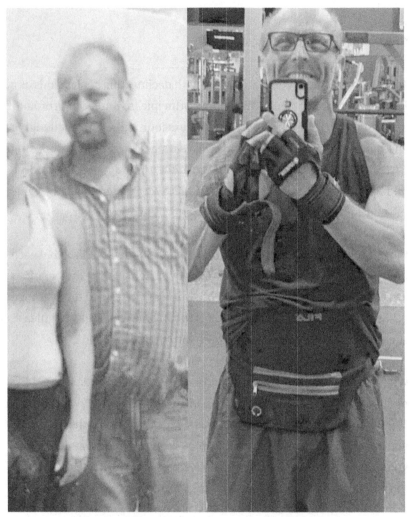

Before– Poor lifestyle choices and bad habits all around.
After–Healthy lifestyle choices. Turning bad habits into good habits.

Scientific Rationale: Why One Hour?

Research underscores the efficacy of concise, focused exercise sessions. Studies reveal that quality trumps quantity, with high-intensity workouts offering substantial benefits for cardiovascular health, muscle strength, and metabolic functional and critical factors that influence aging. The workouts in this book are sculpted around this science, ensuring you gain the maximum benefit from each minute spent. This approach also aligns with the latest guidelines on physical activity for older adults, emphasizing the importance of a balanced regimen that includes strength, flexibility, and aerobic components.

Structuring Your One-Hour Investment

Each workout session is a microcosm of holistic fitness, designed with a deep understanding of the aging body's needs. We start with stretching, laying the groundwork for mobility and injury prevention. The warm-up phase then elevates your heart rate and prepares your muscles for the work ahead. Strength training follows, targeting key muscle groups to build power, support bone health, and boost metabolism. Cardiovascular training is next, fine-tuned to optimize heart health and endurance without overburdening your joints. Finally, the cool down offers your body the necessary space to recover, ensuring you're ready to tackle the day ahead or enjoy a restorative night's sleep.

The Empowerment of Personal Fitness

This book is more than a collection of workouts; it's a journey towards self-empowerment. Fitness in your 40's, 50's, and 60's brings a wealth of benefits, from enhanced mental clarity and emotional balance to a stronger, more resilient body. It's about reclaiming your vitality, pushing past self-imposed limits, and discovering what you're truly capable of. This guide is your companion, offering not just exercises but motivation, inspiration, and the tools to cultivate a mindset geared towards growth and self-improvement.

Building a Community of Age-Defying Athletes

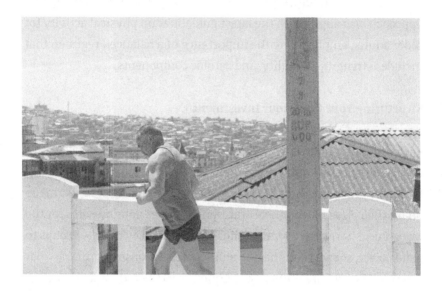

Fitness, at its core, is a personal journey, but it's one that thrives in community. This book aims to unite individuals on similar paths, creating a network of support, encouragement, and shared experience. Through these pages, you'll find stories of transformation, tips from peers, and perhaps a reflection of your own aspirations and challenges. It's a reminder that you're not alone in your quest for health and vitality; there's a vibrant community walking this path with you.

Tailoring the Workout to Your Unique Journey

Recognizing the diversity of experience and ability among athletes in their 40,s, 50,s, and 60,s, this book offers flexibility within its structure. Modifications, alternatives, and progressions are provided, ensuring that whether you're a seasoned marathoner or stepping into the gym for the first time in years, you'll find workouts that challenge and excite you. This adaptability is key, allowing each individual to tailor the program to their needs, goals, and starting point.

A Holistic Approach to Aging and Fitness

As we embark on this journey together, it's essential to view fitness not as a solitary pursuit but as one pillar of a vibrant, healthy life. Nutrition, sleep, stress management, and community engagement are also integral to the aging process. This book embraces a holistic perspective, offering insights and advice that extend beyond the gym, encouraging a lifestyle that supports your fitness goals and overall well being.

2

Getting Started

Embarking on a fitness journey is thrilling, but like any journey, it starts with preparation. This chapter is your starting block, setting you up for success in each one-hour workout. We'll dive into the essentials of a proper warm-up and stretching routine, outline dynamic warm-up exercises tailored for the seasoned athlete, and underscore the critical importance of maintaining form and technique. Let's gear up and set the foundation for a workout that's not only effective but sustainable.

The Foundation: Warm-Up and Stretching

Imagine your body as a classic car. Before hitting the road, you'd warm up the engine, especially on a chilly morning. Similarly, your body needs a gradual transition from rest to activity, preparing your muscles, joints, and cardiovascular system for the workout ahead. A well-executed warm-up enhances performance and, crucially, reduces the risk of injury. It's about showing respect for your body's needs, acknowledging that a little investment upfront pays dividends in safety and effectiveness.

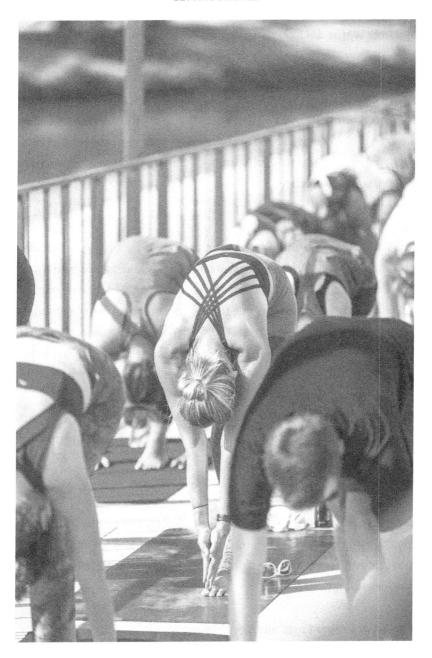

Dynamic Warm-Up Exercises: Movement with Purpose

Gone are the days of static stretching as a pre-workout ritual. Dynamic warm-ups are the order of the day, incorporating movement that not only stretches but also activates your muscles, priming your body for the activities to come. These exercises mirror the workout's intensity but at a lower scale, ensuring a smooth transition. Here's a selection tailored for our audience:

1. Arm Circles: Begin with your arms extended by your sides, gradually making larger circles until you feel your shoulders loosened up.
2. Leg Swings: Hold onto a wall or chair for balance and swing one leg forward and back, then side to side, loosening up your hip flexors and hamstrings.
3. Walking Lunges: Step forward into a lunge, keeping your knee aligned with your ankle. This activates your leg muscles, preparing them for strength training.
4. Torso Twists: With feet shoulder-width apart, gently twist your torso from side to side, engaging your core and warming up your spine.

Each exercise should be performed for about 30 seconds to 1 minute, focusing on fluid, controlled movements. The goal is to increase your heart rate and circulation, making your muscles more elastic and ready for the workout.

The Art of Proper Form and Technique

Maintaining proper form isn't just about effectiveness; it's about safety.

As we age, the margin for error narrows, and the importance of technique becomes paramount. Each exercise in this program is designed with the older athlete in mind, but even the best-designed workout can lead to injury if performed incorrectly.

Here's where mindfulness enters the equation. Approach each exercise with focus, paying attention to your body's alignment and movement. Listen to your body, it's your best coach. If a movement feels wrong, it likely is. Prioritize quality over quantity; it's better to perform fewer repetitions correctly than to rush through them at the expense of your form. Here are key points to remember:

Alignment: Keep your body aligned, especially your spine. Misalignment puts unnecessary stress on your joints and muscles.
Breathing: Never hold your breath. Ensure you're breathing evenly throughout your exercises, oxygenating your muscles and maintaining a steady rhythm.
Control: Movements should be deliberate and controlled, avoiding momentum that can lead to injury. Embrace the full range of motion, but never force it.

Mesocycles: Structuring Your Training Journey

A mesocycle is part of a periodized training plan, typically spanning several weeks, where you focus on a specific training goal. Each mesocycle builds upon the last, allowing for progressive overload and recovery, crucial for athletes of all ages but particularly for those in their 40's, 50's and 60's. Here are the different types of mesocycles:

1. Endurance Mesocycle: Focuses on improving cardiovascular fit-

ness and muscular endurance. Workouts might include longer, moderate-intensity cardio sessions and higher-rep, lower-weight strength training with minimal rest between sets.

2. Strength Mesocycle: Aims to increase overall muscle strength. This phase involves lifting heavier weights with fewer repetitions and includes longer rest periods between sets to allow for muscle recovery.

3. Hypertrophy Mesocycle: Targets muscle growth by focusing on a moderate range of repetitions (typically 6-12) with weights that challenge the muscles, combined with short to moderate rest periods.

4. Power Mesocycle: Focuses on increasing explosive strength and speed. This involves performing exercises at a faster pace or with explosive movements, often using lighter weights or body weight.

5. Recovery Mesocycle: A lighter training phase focusing on active recovery, flexibility, and mobility work to allow the body to recover and prepare for the next cycle of training.

Understanding Body Types

Incorporating the concept of body types, or somatotypes, can further personalize your training and nutritional approach. There are three primary body types:

Endomorphs: Characterized by a higher body fat percentage, endo-morphs tend to gain weight easily and have a rounder body shape. They might find it more challenging to lose fat but can build muscle effectively. For endomorphs, a combination of cardiovascular exercises to aid in fat loss and strength training to build muscle is beneficial.

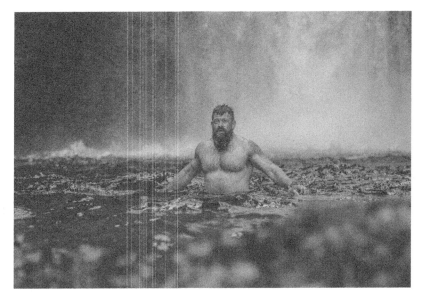

Endomorph

Ectomorphs: Often slim with a fast metabolism, ectomorphs might find it difficult to gain weight and muscle. They have a narrow frame. Ectomorphs can benefit from focusing on hypertrophy and strength mesocycles, with an emphasis on calorie-dense nutrition to support muscle growth.

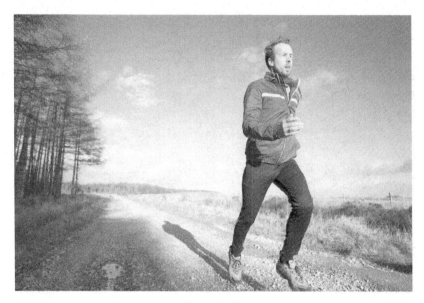

Ectomorph

Mesomorphs: This body type finds it relatively easy to gain and lose weight and can build muscle quickly. They have a naturally athletic physique. Mesomorphs can generally adapt well to any type of training but might focus on balancing their workouts between strength, hypertrophy, and endurance to maintain their physique and fitness levels.

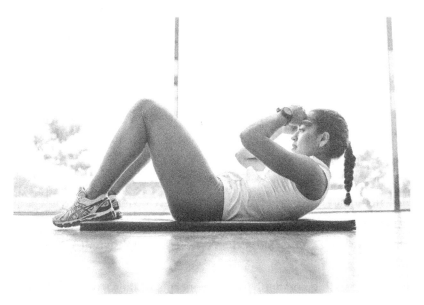

Mesomorph

Applying Mesocycles and Body Types to Your Workouts

For athletes in their 40's, 50's, and 60's, understanding these concepts is vital for creating a workout program that respects their body's capabilities and goals. For instance:

An endomorph might start with an endurance mesocycle to increase cardiovascular health and aid in fat loss, gradually transitioning into strength and hypertrophy cycles to build muscle while continuously incorporating cardio.

An ectomorph, aiming to build muscle mass, might prioritize hypertrophy and strength mesocycles, ensuring adequate calorie intake to support growth, with less emphasis on cardio.

A mesomorph could benefit from a varied approach, alternating between different types of mesocycles to continually challenge their body and improve all aspects of their fitness.

For each body type, the recovery mesocycle becomes increasingly important with age, ensuring adequate time for rest and recuperation to prevent injuries and support longevity in fitness.

(Recent studies have stated that body types are no longer categorized. I do not agree. Genetics play a big part on how our bodies react to physical stimuli. No body type is better than the other, just different.)

By understanding and applying the concepts of mesocycles and body types, athletes in their 40's, 50's, and 60's can more effectively tailor their one-hour workouts to achieve their fitness goals, ensuring they're not just working hard but working smart. This approach fosters a sustainable and enjoyable fitness journey, allowing for personal growth, improved health, and a deeper understanding of one's body and its needs.

Setting the Stage for Success

As we conclude this chapter, remember that a strong start sets the tone for the entire workout. Your warm-up and attention to form are not just preliminary steps; they are integral parts of your fitness journey. They lay the groundwork for a workout that not only achieves its goals but does so in a way that respects and protects your body.

With the foundation laid, we're ready to move forward. The upcoming chapters will delve into specific exercises and routines, but always carry forward the principles of preparation, mindfulness, and respect for your body. Welcome to the heart of your workout journey, where each step is informed, intentional, and geared towards your holistic well-being.

3

Push Exercises

Welcome to the heart of strength training: the push exercises. This chapter is dedicated to sculpting your chest, shoulders, and triceps, and key components of a balanced and powerful upper body. These exercises are designed not only to build strength but also to enhance functional movement, improve posture, and increase your overall metabolic rate. Let's dive into the specifics, ensuring you're equipped to perform each exercise with perfect form and understand how to adapt them to your fitness level.

1. The Classic Push-Up

How to Perform:

1. Start in a plank position, hands slightly wider than shoulder-width apart, body in a straight line from head to heels.
2. Engage your core and glutes, then lower your body until your chest nearly touches the floor, elbows bending at a 45-degree angle to your body.
3. Push through your palms, extending your arms to return to the

starting position.

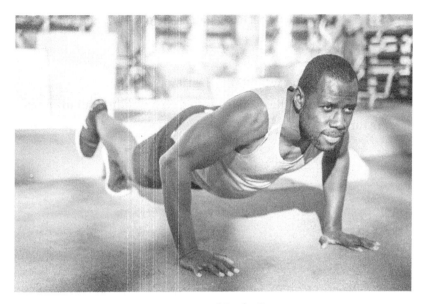

One-Legged Push-Up

Modifications:

Beginner: Perform push-ups on your knees or against a wall to reduce the intensity.

Advanced: Elevate your feet on a bench or step for a decline push-up, increasing the challenge.

2. The Shoulder Press

How to Perform:

1. Stand or sit with your feet shoulder-width apart, holding a dumb-bell in each hand at shoulder height, palms facing forward.
2. Press the weights upward until your arms are fully extended overhead, without locking your elbows.
3. Lower the dumbbells back to shoulder height with control.

Modifications:

Beginner: Use lighter weights or a resistance band.

Advanced: Perform the exercise seated on a stability ball to engage the core further.

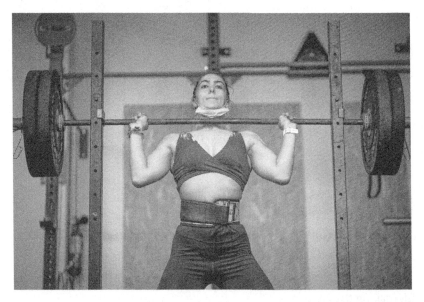

Front Shoulder Press

3. The Bench Press

How to Perform:

1. Lie on a bench with your feet flat on the floor, eyes under the barbell. Grip the bar slightly wider than shoulder-width.
2. Unrack the bar, lowering it to the middle of your chest while keeping your elbows at a 45-degree angle.
3. Press the bar up and away from your chest until your arms are straight, focusing on engaging your chest muscles.

Modifications:

Beginner: Use a smith machine or dumbbells for more stability.

Advanced: Incorporate an incline or decline bench to target different parts of the chest.

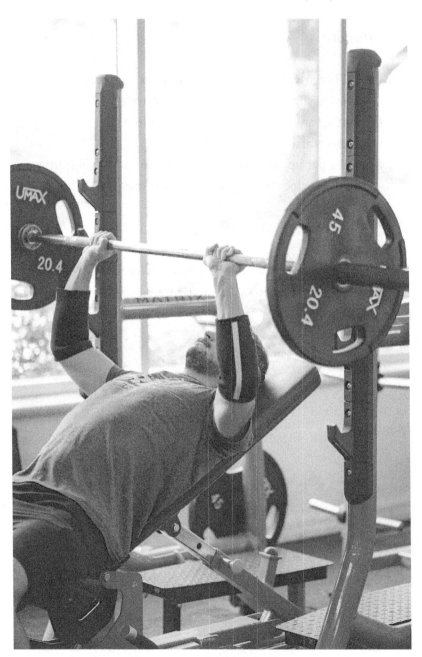

Incline Bench Press

4. Dumbbell Lateral Raises

How to Perform:

1. Stand with feet hip-width apart, holding a dumbbell in each hand at your sides, palms facing in.
2. Keeping a slight bend in your elbows, lift the dumbbells out to your sides until they reach shoulder height, then lower back down with control.

Modifications:

Beginner: Perform one arm at a time to maintain balance and control.

Advanced: Add a slight pause at the top of the movement to increase muscle activation.

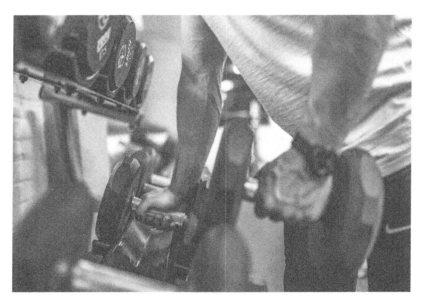

Dumbbells for Lateral Raises

5. Tricep Dips

How to Perform:

1. Sit on the edge of a chair or bench, hands gripping the edge next to your hips, fingers facing forward.
2. Extend your legs out in front of you, then slide your buttocks off the edge, supporting your weight with your arms.
3. Lower your body by bending your elbows to a 90-degree angle, then press back up to the starting position.

Modifications:

Beginner: Bend your knees to reduce the load on your triceps.

Advanced: Elevate your feet on another bench or add weight to your lap to increase resistance.

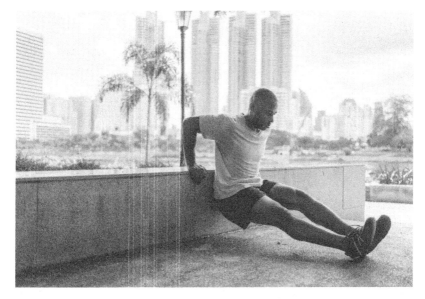

Seated Tricep Dip

Embracing Your Workout

Each exercise within this push workout is designed to challenge and grow your upper body's strength, offering versatility to accommodate various fitness levels and physical limitations. Remember, the key to progress is consistency, proper form, and gradually increasing the challenge as your strength improves.

As you integrate these push exercises into your one-hour workouts, listen to your body, focusing on quality over quantity. With dedication and patience, you'll build a strong, functional upper body capable of tackling both everyday activities and athletic endeavors with ease.

4

Pull Exercises

I n the symphony of strength training, if push exercises are the melody, pull exercises are the harmony. This chapter zooms in on the pull movements that target your back, biceps, and forearms. Pull exercises are crucial for creating a balanced physique, improving posture, and enhancing overall upper body strength. Let's explore a variety of pull exercises, ensuring you know how to execute them safely and effectively, with modifications to cater to all fitness levels.

1. The Bent-Over Row

How to Perform:

1. Stand with feet shoulder-width apart, knees slightly bent, and hold a barbell or dumbbells in front of you.
2. Hinge at your hips to lean forward, keeping your back straight, and let the weights hang directly in front of you.
3. Pull the weights towards your lower ribs, squeezing your shoulder blades together. Lower them back down with control.

Modifications:

Beginner: Use light dumbbells or a resistance band.

Advanced: Perform the exercise on one leg to engage the core and improve balance.

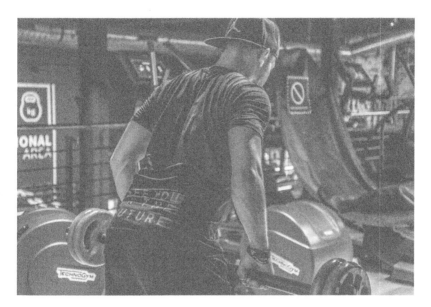

Bent-Over Row

2. The Pull-Up

How to Perform:

1. Grip a pull-up bar with your hands slightly wider than shoulder-width apart, palms facing away from you.
2. Hang with your arms fully extended, then pull yourself up until

your chin is above the bar.

3. Lower yourself back down slowly to the full hang position.

Modifications:

Beginner: Use an assisted pull-up machine or resistance bands for support.

Advanced: Add weight with a belt or hold a dumbbell between your feet.

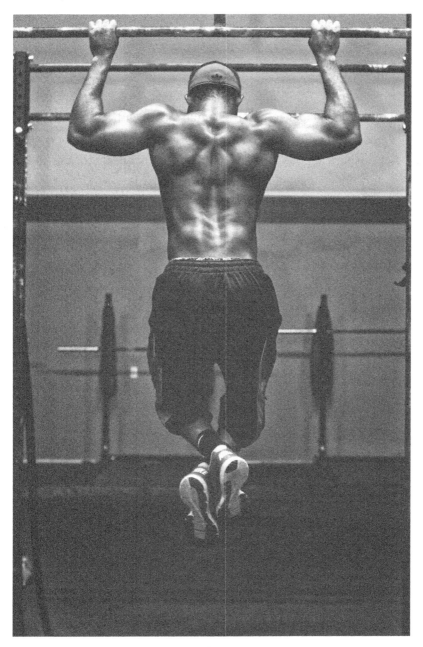

Pull Up

3. The Lat Pulldown

How to Perform:

1. Sit at a lat pulldown station and grab the bar with an overhand grip, hands wider than shoulder width.
2. Lean back slightly, chest up, and pull the bar down to your chest, drawing your shoulder blades down and back.
3. Slowly return the bar to the starting position, controlling the weight through the ascent.

Modifications:

Beginner: Start with lighter weight to focus on form and technique.

Advanced: Use a wide grip or a close reverse grip to target the muscles differently.

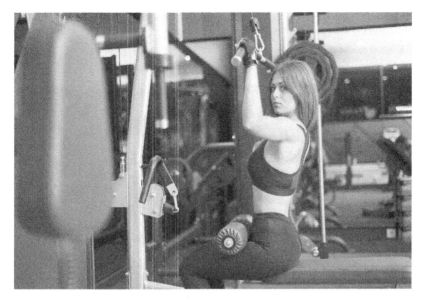

Cable Lat Pulldown

4. Seated Cable Row

How to Perform:

1. Sit at a cable row machine with your feet braced and knees slightly bent.
2. Grab the handle with both hands, keeping your back straight and shoulders down.
3. Pull the handle towards your abdomen, squeezing your shoulder blades together. Extend your arms to return to the starting position.

Modifications:

Beginner: Focus on light weight and perfecting the movement pattern.

Advanced: Try a single-arm version to isolate each side of your back

31

and correct imbalances.

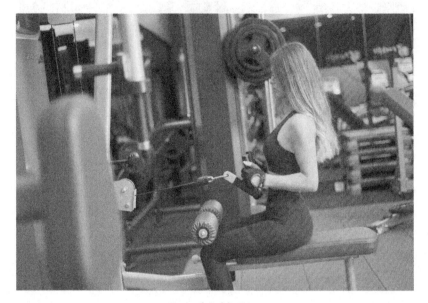

Seated Cable Row

5. Bicep Curls

How to Perform:

1. Stand with feet hip-width apart, holding dumbbells at your sides with palms facing forward.
2. Keeping your elbows close to your torso, curl the weights towards your shoulders, contracting your biceps.
3. Lower the weights back down with control to the starting position.
4. Modifications:

Beginner: Use light weights or a resistance band.

Advanced: Perform the exercise standing on one leg to engage the core, or try hammer curls for variation.

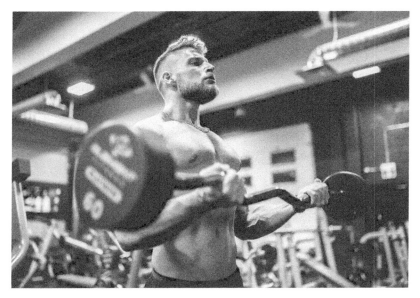

Easy-Bar Curls

Pulling It All Together

Pull exercises are essential for building a strong, functional back and upper body. They help counteract the effects of daily activities that may contribute to poor posture by strengthening the muscles responsible for pulling actions. By incorporating these exercises into your routine, you'll not only enhance your physical appearance but also improve your functional abilities in everyday life and athletic performance.

Remember, progression is key. Start with modifications suited to your current fitness level and gradually increase the intensity as your strength and confidence grow. Pay close attention to your form, ensuring each movement is performed with precision and control. With consistency and dedication, you'll notice significant improvements in your strength, posture, and overall well-being.

5

Leg Exercises

Building a foundation of strength, stability, and power starts from the ground up, with your legs. This chapter is dedicated to sculpting strong, resilient legs that support not just your fitness goals but your day-to-day life. We'll focus on exercises targeting the quadriceps, hamstrings, glutes, and calves, ensuring a well-rounded leg workout. Proper form and technique are paramount to maximize benefits and minimize the risk of injury, especially for those with knee or hip limitations.

1. Squats

How to Perform:

1. Stand with feet shoulder-width apart, toes slightly turned out.
2. Keeping your chest up and back straight, lower into a squat by bending at the knees and hips, as if sitting back into a chair.
3. Lower down until your thighs are parallel to the floor (or as low as comfortable), then drive through your heels to return to standing.

Modifications:

Knee Limitations: Perform box squats by squatting to a bench or chair, limiting the depth to avoid knee pain.

Advanced: Add weight with dumbbells, a barbell, or a kettlebell to increase intensity.

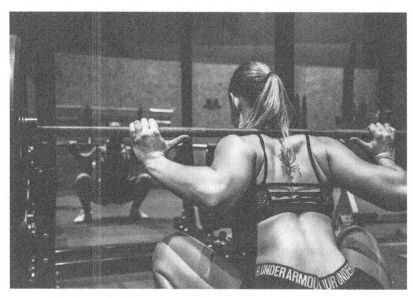

Back Squat

2. Lunges

How to Perform:

1. Start in a standing position, step forward with one leg, and lower your hips until both knees are bent at about a 90-degree angle.

36

2. Make sure your front knee is directly above your ankle and your back knee hovers just above the floor.

3. Push back up to the starting position through the heel of your front foot.

Modifications:

Knee Limitations: Reduce the depth of the lunge or perform a reverse lunge, stepping backward instead of forward, to reduce stress on the knees.

Advanced: Hold dumbbells in each hand to add resistance or perform walking lunges for added difficulty and dynamic balance.

3. Deadlifts

How to Perform:

1. Stand with feet hip-width apart, a barbell or dumbbells in front of your thighs.

2. Hinge at the hips to lower the weights toward the ground, keeping your back flat and chest up.

3. Push through your heels to return to standing, driving the hips forward to engage the glutes and hamstrings.

Modifications:

Hip Limitations: Try a Romanian deadlift with a slight bend in the knees, focusing on hip hinge movement to reduce strain.

Advanced: Increase the weight as you become more comfortable with the form, or try single-leg deadlifts to challenge balance and unilateral strength.

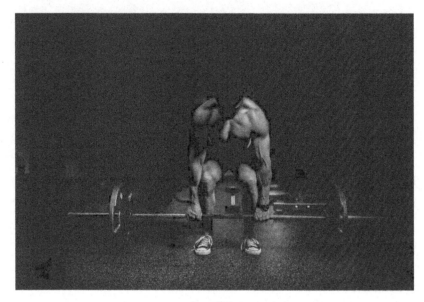

Deadlifts

4. Calf Raises

How to Perform:

1. Stand upright, feet hip-width apart, holding onto a wall or chair for balance if needed.
2. Lift your heels off the ground, rising onto your toes, then slowly lower back down.
3. For added intensity, perform the exercise on a step or ledge, allowing your heels to drop below the level of your toes before pushing up.

Modifications:
Knee Limitations: Perform the movement slowly and with control to

minimize impact on the knees.

Advanced: Hold weights for added resistance or perform single-leg calf raises to increase the challenge.

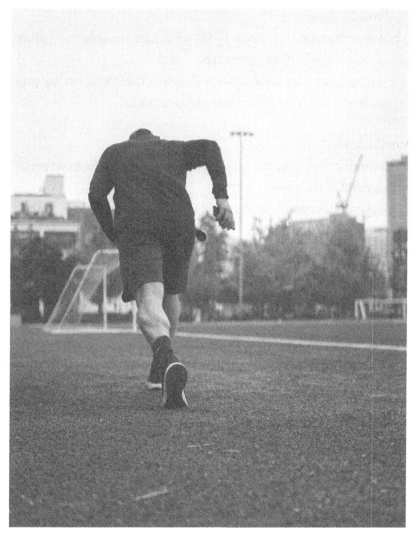

Gastrocnemius (calf) Muscle

5. Glute Bridges

How to Perform:

1. Lie on your back with knees bent and feet flat on the floor, close to your buttocks.
2. Press through your heels to lift your hips towards the ceiling, squeezing your glutes at the top.
3. Lower your hips back down with control, without letting your buttocks touch the floor between repetitions.

Modifications:

Hip Limitations: Keep the range of motion small and focus on gentle engagement of the glutes.

Advanced: Place a weight on your hips for added resistance or perform the exercise with one leg lifted off the ground to target each side more intensely.

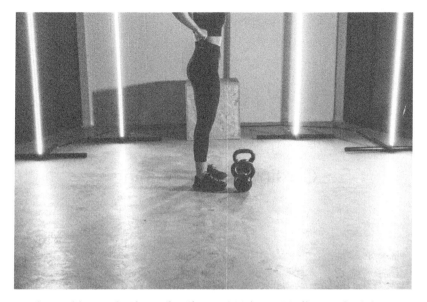

Glute Bridges Help Shape the Gluteus Maximus, Medius, and Minimus.

Building Your Leg Day Foundation

These exercises form the core of a comprehensive leg workout, aiming to improve strength, flexibility, and endurance in the lower body. Remember, adjusting each exercise to fit your current fitness level and any limitations is crucial for safe and effective training. Consistency, proper form, and gradual progression are key to unlocking the full potential of your leg workouts. As you develop strength and confidence, feel free to explore more advanced variations and additional weight to keep challenging your lower body.

6

Cardiovascular Training

I n the quest for a balanced fitness regimen, cardiovascular training stands as a cornerstone, essential for not just physical health but overall well-being. This chapter delves into the heart of cardio exercises-pun intended-highlighting their significance, especially for athletes in their 40's, 50's, and 60's. We'll explore a variety of cardio workouts that are both effective and accommodating to the mature athlete, along with strategies to seamlessly weave them into your one-hour workout routine.

The Heart of the Matter: Why Cardio Matters

Cardiovascular exercise, also known as aerobic exercise, involves sustained physical activity that increases your heart rate and blood circulation. Its benefits are manifold: improved heart health, increased lung capacity, reduced risk of chronic diseases, enhanced mood and mental health, and effective weight management. For the older athlete, cardio adds another layer of advantage by helping maintain mobility, balance, and endurance, ensuring that you can enjoy an active, vibrant lifestyle for years to come.

Cardio Options for the Mature Athlete

1. **Walking**: The most accessible form of cardio, walking can be surprisingly effective. It's low-impact, can be done anywhere, and easily adjusted in intensity. Consider brisk walking, hill walks, or Nordic walking to up the challenge.
2. **Cycling**: Whether outdoors or on a stationary bike, cycling is excellent for cardiovascular fitness without the high impact on your joints. It's also a fantastic way to build leg strength and endurance
3. **Swimming**: A total body workout that's gentle on the body, swimming is ideal for those with joint concerns or those looking for a soothing yet effective cardio session. It improves not only your heart health but also your muscle strength and flexibility.
4. **Rowing**: An often-overlooked cardio workout, rowing on a machine provides a low-impact, full-body exercise that enhances both cardiovascular fitness and muscle endurance.
5. **Dance or Aerobic Classes**: Joining a dance or aerobic class can be a fun and social way to get your cardio in. These activities are scalable to your fitness level and can be highly motivating.

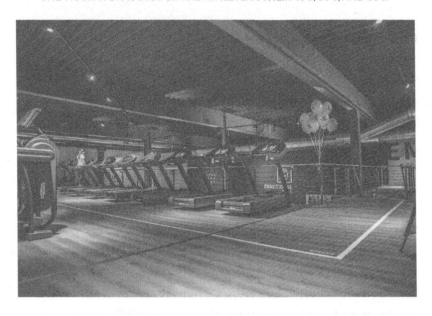

Incorporating Cardio into Your One-Hour Routine

To make the most out of your one-hour workout, consider the following strategies for integrating cardiovascular training:

Warm-Up with Purpose: Start your session with a 10-minute moderate-intensity cardio warm-up. This could be a brisk walk or a gentle cycle, setting the stage for the rest of your workout.

High-Intensity Interval Training (HIIT): If you're pressed for time but want to maximize your cardio benefits, include short bursts of high-intensity exercises followed by brief recovery periods. For example, 1 minute of intense cycling followed by 2 minutes of lighter pedaling, repeated for 15-20 minutes, can be incredibly effective.

Split Your Sessions: Consider dedicating specific days to focused cardio training, alternating with strength training days. This approach allows you to target different aspects of fitness without overwhelming your body.

Cool Down with Cardio: End your workout with a 5-10 minute low-intensity cardio cool-down. This helps in recovery by gradually lowering your heart rate and preventing blood from pooling in your extremities.

Listen to Your Body: The key to successful cardiovascular training is to listen to your body and adjust accordingly. If you're feeling fatigued, opt for lower-intensity options. Conversely, challenge yourself with higher intensities as your fitness improves.

Creating a Balanced Approach

Cardiovascular training is more than just a means to an end; it's a way to enrich your life, enhance your health, and enjoy the activities you love with vigor and vitality. By thoughtfully incorporating cardio into your one-hour workouts, you're not just working towards a fitter body but also ensuring a healthier, more dynamic life in your 40's, 50's, and beyond. Remember, consistency is key, and every step, pedal, or stroke takes you closer to your fitness goals.

7

Stretching and Flexibility

A s we navigate through our fitness journey, especially in our 40's, 50's, and 60's, the importance of stretching and flexibility cannot be overstated. This chapter is dedicated to the art and science of stretching, a critical component of any comprehensive workout routine. Stretching not only aids in injury prevention but also enhances joint mobility, allowing for a more fluid, pain-free range of motion. Let's explore effective stretching exercises and the added benefits of incorporating disciplines like yoga and Pilates into your regimen.

The Foundation of Flexibility

Flexibility training involves two primary types of stretching: dynamic and static.

Dynamic stretches are performed as part of your warm-up, using controlled movements to prepare your muscles and joints for the workout ahead. Static stretches, on the other hand, are done post-workout, holding a stretch position for a longer period to improve flexibility and relax your muscles.

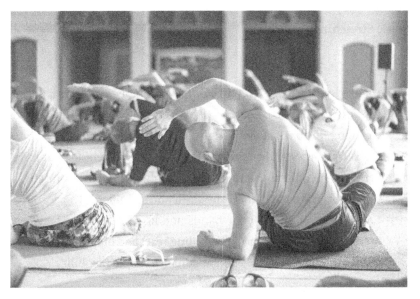

Stretching for Flexibility.

Dynamic Stretching Exercises

1. Arm Circles: Extend your arms to the sides and rotate them in small circles, gradually increasing the size. This warms up the shoulders and arms.
2. Leg Swings: Hold onto a stable surface for support and swing one leg forward and back, then side to side. This loosens up the hips, hamstrings, and quadriceps.
3. Walking Lunges with a Twist: Perform a forward lunge and gently twist your torso towards the front leg. This activates the lower body and stretches the spine and abdominals.

Static Stretching Exercises

1. Hamstring Stretch: Sit on the floor with your legs extended. Reach towards your toes, keeping your knees straight but not locked. Hold to stretch the back of your thighs.
2. Chest Opener: Stand or sit and clasp your hands behind your back. Straighten your arms and lift them slightly, opening your chest. This stretch is excellent for the chest and shoulders.
3. Cat-Cow Stretch: On your hands and knees, alternate between arching your back towards the ceiling (cat) and dipping it towards the floor (cow). This movement enhances spine flexibility.

Incorporating Yoga and Pilates

Beyond individual stretches, integrating yoga or Pilates into your workout routine offers profound benefits for flexibility, strength, and mental well-being.

Yoga: Combines physical postures, breathing techniques, and meditation to enhance flexibility, muscle tone, and stress relief. Yoga practices range from gentle to challenging, accommodating all fitness levels. Poses like the Downward Dog, Warrior series, and Pigeon pose are excellent for building flexibility and strength.

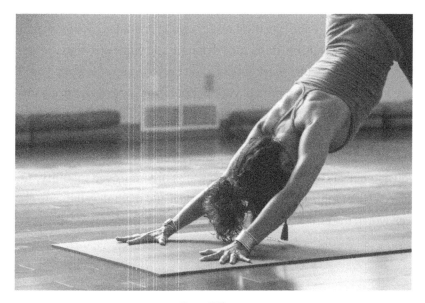

Yoga/Pilates

Pilates: Focuses on core strength, posture, balance, and flexibility. Through controlled movements and breathing, Pilates exercises strengthen the body's "powerhouse" the abdominals, lower back, hips, and buttocks. Incorporating Pilates into your routine can improve joint mobility and stability, particularly beneficial as we age.

Embracing Flexibility in Your Routine

Dedicating time to stretching and flexibility exercises is essential for maintaining a healthy, active lifestyle as you age. It's not just about preventing injuries; it's about enhancing your quality of life, ensuring that you can continue to perform daily activities and enjoy your favorite hobbies without pain or restriction.

Consider setting aside specific days for a yoga or Pilates session as part of your weekly routine, or include dynamic and static stretches before and after your regular workouts. As you become more flexible, you'll likely notice improvements in your overall fitness performance and a reduction in discomforts associated with tight muscles and stiff joints.

Remember, flexibility training is a journey, not a destination. It requires consistency and patience, but the rewards are improved mobility, reduced risk of injury, and enhanced physical and mental well-being are well worth the effort.

8

Cool down and Recovery

As we conclude each workout, it's crucial not to overlook the final act, the cool down and recovery phase. This chapter emphasizes the significance of gradually lowering your body's intensity after exercise and adopting practices that foster recovery. Understanding the importance of this phase can enhance your overall fitness experience, aiding in muscle relaxation, injury prevention, and preparing your body for the next training session.

The Art of Cooling Down

A proper cool down serves as a bridge between the end of your workout and the return to a state of rest. It helps to gradually reduce your heart rate and breathing, minimize muscle stiffness, and start the recovery process. Here's how to effectively integrate a cool down into your routine:

1. Gradual Decrease in Intensity: Begin by reducing the intensity of your workout. If you've been running, shift to a brisk walk,

gradually slowing to a comfortable pace.

2. Static Stretching: Once your heart rate has started to come down, engage in static stretching, focusing on major muscle groups used during your workout. Hold each stretch for 15-30 seconds, breathing deeply to assist in relaxation and flexibility. Include stretches for your hamstrings, quadriceps, calves, chest, back, and shoulders.

3. Deep Breathing: Incorporate deep breathing exercises to calm the nervous system and reduce stress. Sit or lie down comfortably, inhale deeply through the nose, hold for a few seconds, and exhale slowly through the mouth. Repeat several times.

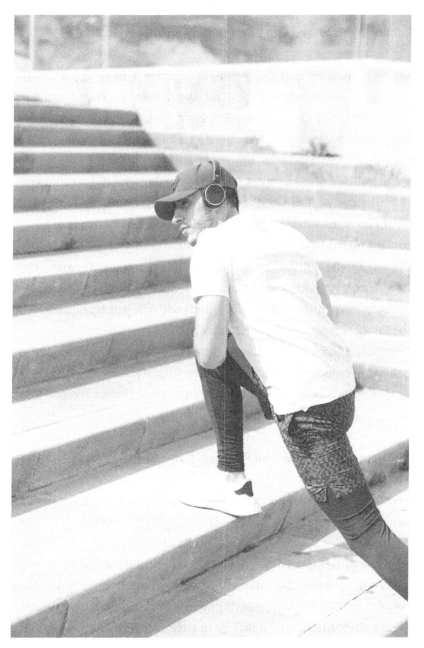

Static Stretching

Enhancing Recovery with Foam Rolling and Recovery Tools

Recovery tools such as foam rollers, massage balls, and percussion massagers can significantly enhance your post-workout routine by improving blood circulation, releasing muscle tightness, and aiding in the breakdown of soft tissue adhesions known as "knots."

Foam Rolling: Also known as self-myofascial release, foam rolling can be particularly effective for areas prone to tightness, such as the IT band, calves, hamstrings, and back. Roll slowly over each muscle group, pausing on tender spots for 15-30 seconds.

Massage Balls: These can target smaller, more specific areas that are difficult to reach with a foam roller, such as the feet, glutes, and shoulders. Apply pressure to the muscle with the ball against a wall or the floor and gently move back and forth.

Percussion Massagers: These devices offer deep tissue stimulation, helping to reduce soreness and improve mobility. Use them on various muscle groups, adjusting the intensity according to your comfort level.

The Benefits of a Dedicated Recovery Strategy

Investing time in cool down and recovery practices can offer numerous benefits:

Reduced Muscle Soreness: Gentle stretching and the use of recovery tools can alleviate the intensity of delayed onset muscle soreness (DOMS), making the days following intense workouts more comfortable.

Injury Prevention: By aiding in muscle recovery and maintaining flexibility, you're less likely to suffer injuries that can arise from over-training or muscle imbalances. **Improved Performance**: Recovery is when your body repairs and strengthens itself. Adequate recovery not only prevents burnout but also sets the stage for better performance in future workouts.

Incorporating Cool down and Recovery into Your Routine

To maximize the benefits of your fitness regimen, treat cool down and recovery with the same importance as the workout itself. Dedicate at least 5-10 minutes after every session to a structured cool down, followed by a focus on recovery techniques that suit your body's needs. Remember, recovery is not just a process but an essential component of your fitness journey, ensuring longevity and enjoyment in your activities well into your 40's, 50's, and beyond.

9

Weekly Workout Plans

C rafting a balanced weekly workout plan is key to achieving comprehensive fitness, especially for athletes in their 40's, 50's, and 60's. This chapter provides structured weekly routines that blend push, pull, and leg exercises with cardiovascular training and flexibility work. Tailored for different fitness levels, these plans ensure progress and adaptation over time, all within a one-hour daily workout framework.

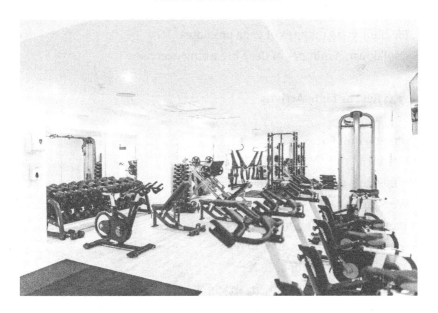

Beginner Level Plan

Day 1: Full Body Strength

Warm-Up: 5 minutes brisk walking or cycling
  Workout:
  Squats: 2 sets of 8-10 reps
  Push-Ups (on knees if necessary): 2 sets of 8-10 reps
  Bent-Over Row with Dumbbells: 2 sets of 8-10 reps
  Cardio: 20 minutes moderate-intensity cycling
  Cool down: 5 minutes of stretching focusing on major muscle groups

Day 2: Cardio & Flexibility

Warm-Up: 5 minutes of dynamic stretching
  Cardio: 30 minutes of brisk walking

Flexibility: 20 minutes of yoga or Pilates

Cool down: 5 minutes of deep breathing exercises

Day 3: Rest or Light Activity

4: Push & Pull Focus

Warm-Up: 5 minutes of light jogging

Workout:

Dumbbell Shoulder Press: 2 sets of 8-10 reps

Lat Pull down: 2 sets of 8-10 reps

Tricep Dips: 2 sets of 8-10 reps

Cardio: 15 minutes of rowing machine

Cool down: 5 minutes of stretching focusing on arms and back

Day 5: Leg Focus & Core

Warm-Up: 5 minutes of dynamic leg stretches

Workout:

Lunges: 2 sets of 8-10 reps per leg

Glute Bridges: 2 sets of 12 reps

Plank: Hold for 30 seconds, repeat twice

Cardio: 20 minutes of low-impact aerobic exercise (e.g., swimming)

Cool down: 5 minutes of full-body stretching

Day 6: Active Recovery

Participate in a light activity you enjoy, such as a leisurely bike ride, swimming, or a nature walk.

Day 7: Rest

(Our bodies are made to do work. We really do not need to take a day off. If you feel you need a rest day, take it. I do. On rest days, I make them **Active Recovery** days.)

Advanced Level Plan

Day 1: Push Focus

Warm-Up: 10 minutes of dynamic stretching and light cardio
  Workout:
  Bench Press: 3 sets of 8-12 reps
  Overhead Dumbbell Press: 3 sets of 8-12 reps
  Push-Ups: 3 sets to failure
  Cardio: 10 minutes HIIT on stationary bike
  Cool down: 10 minutes of static stretching

Day 2: Pull Focus

Warm-Up: 10 minutes rowing
  Workout:
  Deadlifts: 3 sets of 8-10 reps
  Pull-Ups or Assisted Pull-Ups: 3 sets of 6-8 reps
  Seated Cable Row: 3 sets of 8-12 reps
  Cardio: 15 minutes of steady-state jogging or elliptical
  Cool down: 10 minutes of stretching, focusing on back and biceps

Day 3: Cardio & Core

Warm-Up: 5 minutes of dynamic stretching
  Cardio: 30 minutes of mixed cardio (cycling, jogging, rowing)
  Core:

Russian Twists: 3 sets of 15 reps per side

Leg Raises: 3 sets of 10 reps

Cool down: 10 minutes of yoga or Pilates focusing on flexibility

Day 4: Rest or Light Activity

Day 5: Leg & Glute Focus

Warm-Up: 10 minutes of light jogging and dynamic leg stretches

Workout:

Squats (with weight): 3 sets of 8-12 reps

Walking Lunges (holding dumbbells): 3 sets of 10 reps per leg

Calf Raises: 3 sets of 15 reps

Cardio: 10 minutes of HIIT (sprint intervals)

Cool down: 10 minutes of stretching focusing on legs and glutes

Day 6: Full Body Circuit

Warm-Up: 10 minutes of mixed cardio (cycling, jogging)

Circuit (Repeat 3x):

10 Dumbbell Squats

10 Push-Ups

Day 7: Rest

10

Nutrition and Supplement Tips

Nutrition and hydration play pivotal roles in optimizing performance, enhancing recovery, and supporting the overall health of athletes, especially as we age. This chapter will delve into the principles of a balanced diet tailored for the mature athlete and explore supplements that can complement your fitness journey, ensuring you have the energy and resilience to meet your training demands.

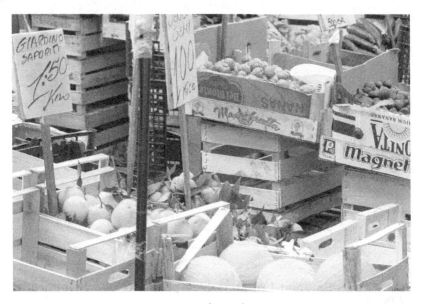

Farmer's Market

Fueling Performance and Recovery Through Nutrition

A balanced diet is your foundation for maintaining energy levels, achieving fitness goals, and recovering effectively from workouts. Here's how to structure your nutrition to support your athletic endeavors:

Macronutrients:
Proteins: Essential for muscle repair and growth. Include lean sources like chicken, fish, tofu, legumes, and dairy in your meals.
Carbohydrates: Your primary energy source. Opt for complex carbs such as whole grains, fruits, and vegetables to maintain stable blood sugar levels.
Fats: Necessary for hormone production and nutrient absorption. Focus on healthy fats found in avocados, nuts, seeds, and olive oil.

Micronutrients:

Pay attention to micronutrients that are crucial for aging athletes, such as calcium, vitamin D, magnesium, and omega-3 fatty acids, to support bone health, reduce inflammation, and enhance heart health.

Hydration:

Adequate water intake is vital for optimal physiological function and performance. Aim for at least 8-10 glasses of water a day, more if you're active or in hot climates. Hydration supports joint lubrication, temperature regulation, and nutrient transport.

Dietary Guidelines for Older Athletes

Frequent, Balanced Meals: Consume smaller, nutrient-dense meals throughout the day to sustain energy and facilitate muscle repair. Include a balance of proteins, carbohydrates, and fats in each meal.

Antioxidant-Rich Foods: Incorporate plenty of fruits and vegetables to combat oxidative stress and support immune function. Berries, leafy greens, and brightly colored vegetables are excellent choices.

Adequate Protein Intake: Aim for 1.2 to 2.0 grams of protein per kilogram of body weight daily to support muscle maintenance and growth, especially important as muscle mass tends to decline with age. Remember to convert your weight into kilograms when aiming for your protein goals. Aim for 0.5 to 0.7 grams of protein per pound of body weight.

Supplements for the Aging Athlete

While whole foods should always be the priority, certain supplements can offer additional benefits:

Protein Powders (Whey, Casein, or Plant-Based): Convenient for ensuring adequate protein intake, especially post-workout for muscle recovery.

Omega-3 Fatty Acids (Fish Oil): Beneficial for heart health, joint mobility, and reducing inflammation.

Vitamin D and Calcium: Important for bone health, particularly for those at risk of osteoporosis or with limited sun exposure.

B Vitamins: Support energy production and red blood cell formation. B12 is particularly important as absorption can decrease with age.

Creatine: Can enhance strength, muscle mass, and recovery, showing benefits in older adults even at low doses.

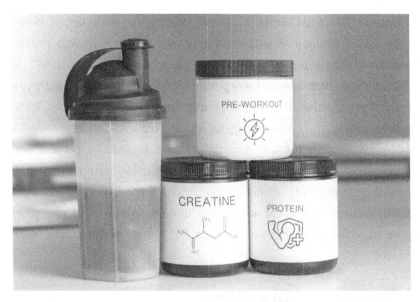

Exercise Supplements

Implementing Nutrition and Supplement Strategies

Incorporating these nutrition and supplement tips into your lifestyle requires planning and consistency. Start by assessing your current diet and identifying areas for improvement. Gradually introduce changes to your eating habits, focusing on whole, unprocessed foods and balanced meals. For supplements, consider consulting with a healthcare provider to ensure they're appropriate for your health status and fitness goals.

Remember, nutrition and hydration are as integral to your fitness success as your workout routine. By nourishing your body with the right foods and supplements, you'll be better equipped to tackle your fitness challenges, recover more effectively, and enjoy a healthier, more active lifestyle at any age.

11

Injury Prevention and Rehabilitations

As athletes progress into their 40's, 50's, and 60's, the risk of injury can increase due to factors like decreased muscle mass, reduced flexibility, and the cumulative impact of wear and tear on the joints. However, with the right precautions and strategies, many common injuries can be prevented, and effective rehabilitation can ensure a swift return to activity. This chapter focuses on addressing these concerns, offering practical advice for maintaining your fitness journey safely.

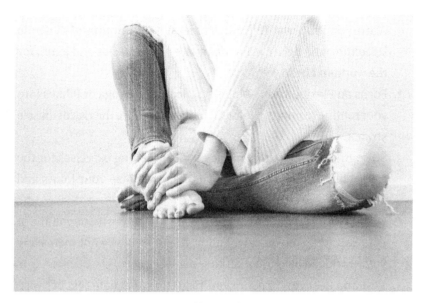

Ankle Sprain

Common Injuries and Issues

Muscle Strains and Sprains: Often occur due to overuse, insufficient warm-up, or a lack of flexibility.

Joint Issues (e.g., Arthritis, Tendinitis): Can result from years of activity, leading to pain and stiffness, particularly in the knees, shoulders, and elbows.

Back Pain: Common due to weakened core muscles or poor posture during exercises.

Rotator Cuff Injuries: Frequent in athletes due to repetitive arm movements.

Injury Prevention Tips

1. Warm-Up Properly: Engage in at least 5-10 minutes of dynamic stretching and light cardio to prepare your muscles and joints for the workout ahead.
2. Focus on Flexibility and Mobility: Incorporate yoga or Pilates into your routine to improve joint mobility and reduce the risk of muscle strains.
3. Strengthen Supporting Muscles: Strengthening exercises for the core, glutes, and leg muscles can help stabilize your joints and prevent injuries.
4. Gradual Progression: Avoid increasing the intensity or volume of your workouts too quickly. Follow the 10% rule by not increasing your workload by more than 10% per week.
5. Rest and Recovery: Ensure you're getting adequate rest between workouts to allow your body to recover and repair itself.

Rehabilitation Exercises

If you do suffer an injury, specific rehabilitation exercises can aid in your recovery. Always consult with a healthcare professional before starting any rehabilitation exercises.

Rotator Cuff Injury: Shoulder external rotation exercises using a resistance band can help strengthen the muscles around the shoulder.
Knee Pain (e.g., from Arthritis or Tendinitis): Leg lifts, hamstring curls, and straight-leg raises can strengthen the muscles supporting your knee without putting excessive strain on it.
Back Pain: Gentle core strengthening exercises like pelvic tilts, bird-dogs, and bridges can support the lower back.
Ankle Sprain: Balance and proprioception exercises, such as standing on one foot or using a balance board, can help restore stability and prevent

future sprains.

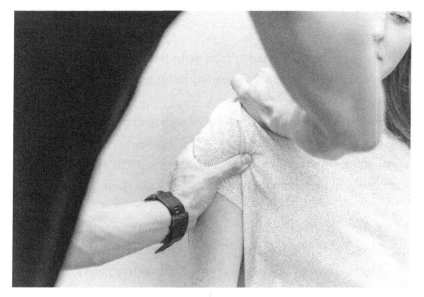

Rotator Cuff Injury

When to Seek Professional Help

It's crucial to listen to your body and recognize when an injury requires professional attention. Seek medical advice if:

1. Pain persists or worsens after a few days of rest and home treatment.
2. You experience severe pain, swelling, numbness, or an inability to bear weight on the affected area.
3. The injured area looks deformed or exhibits signs of infection (e.g., redness, warmth).

69

Modifying Workouts During Recovery

Recovery doesn't mean complete cessation of activity. Modify your workouts by:

1. Focusing on exercises that don't strain the injured area. For example, if you have a lower body injury, you can still engage in upper body strength training.
2. Reducing the intensity and volume of your workouts to avoid further stress on the body.
3. Incorporating more low-impact activities, such as swimming or cycling, which can maintain fitness without exacerbating injuries.

Injury prevention and rehabilitation are key components of a sustainable fitness regimen, particularly for athletes in their later years. By adopting preventative measures, responding appropriately to injuries, and making informed modifications to your workouts, you can enjoy an active, fulfilling lifestyle while minimizing the risk of injury.

12

Motivation and Mindset

E mbarking on and sustaining a fitness journey, especially in the later stages of life, is as much about nurturing a resilient mindset as it is about physical training. This chapter delves into the critical role that motivation and a positive outlook play in achieving and maintaining fitness goals. We'll explore strategies to navigate challenges and setbacks and draw inspiration from older athletes who exemplify what it means to age with strength and grace.

The Foundation of Success: A Positive Mindset

A positive mindset is the bedrock upon which all successful fitness journeys are built. It's about seeing challenges as opportunities for growth, setbacks as temporary, and believing in your ability to achieve your goals. A positive outlook not only enhances your motivation but can also improve your physical performance and recovery.

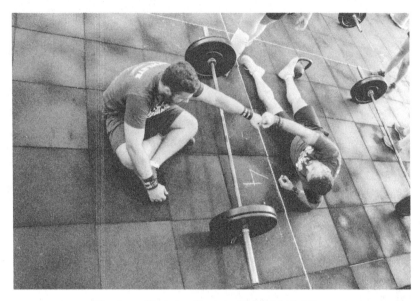

Having a Training Partner Helps Motivation.

Staying Motivated: Strategies for Success

1. Set Clear, Achievable Goals: Break your larger goals into smaller, measurable milestones. Celebrating these victories can fuel your motivation and provide a clear sense of progress.
2. Find Your Why: Identify the deeper reasons behind your fitness journey. Whether it's improving your health, being active with your grandchildren, or challenging yourself, your "why" can be a powerful motivator.
3. Create a Supportive Community: Surround yourself with like-minded individuals who share your fitness goals. Joining a group or finding a workout buddy can provide encouragement, accountability, and a sense of belonging.

4. Embrace Variety: Keep your routine interesting by trying new activities or workouts. This not only prevents boredom but can also lead to new challenges and achievements.

5. Reflect on Your Journey: Regularly take time to reflect on how far you've come. Recognize the effort you've put in and how it has impacted your life positively.

Overcoming Challenges and Setbacks

Challenges and setbacks are inevitable, but they don't define your journey. Here's how to navigate them:

Adopt a Growth Mindset: View setbacks as opportunities to learn and grow. Analyze what happened and how you can adjust your approach moving forward.

Be Kind to Yourself: Practice self-compassion. Remind yourself that progress is not linear and that perseverance is key.

Adjust Your Plan as Needed: Be flexible and willing to modify your goals or approach if circumstances change. Fitness is a lifelong journey, and adaptability is a strength.

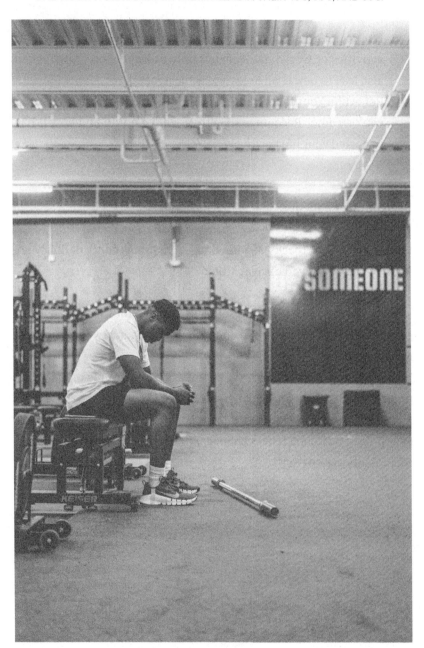

Growth Mindset

Inspirational Stories and Quotes

Let's draw inspiration from those who have shown that age is not a barrier to achieving remarkable fitness goals:

Fauja Singh, who became the first centenarian to complete a marathon, famously said, "The first 20 miles are not difficult. As for the last six miles, I run while talking to God."

Ernestine Shepherd, the world's oldest female bodybuilder, encourages others with her mantra, "Age is nothing but a number.".
Yuichiro Miura, who climbed Mount Everest at the age of 80, shared, "It is important to have some adventures in life."

These stories and quotes remind us that with determination, a positive mindset, and a love for what we do, achieving our fitness goals is possible at any age.

Cultivating a Resilient Mindset

Your fitness journey is uniquely yours, but the principles of motivation, mindset, and perseverance are universal. By fostering a positive outlook, staying motivated through challenges, and drawing inspiration from those who've paved the way, you're not just working towards physical goals but also nurturing a resilient spirit that will carry you through all aspects of life. Remember, it's never too late to set new goals or dream a new dream...

13

Exercise and Diabetes Management: Unlocking the Benefits

For individuals living with diabetes, integrating exercise into daily life is not just beneficial; it's transformative. This chapter delves into the profound impact of physical activity on diabetes management, highlighting the pivotal role of the GLUT4 transporter and examining insulin's anabolic effects compared to testosterone. Understanding these mechanisms can empower those with diabetes to significantly enhance their health and quality of life.

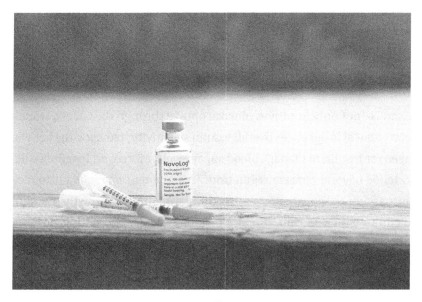

Insulin

The Critical Role of the GLUT4 Transporter in Glucose Metabolism

Central to the benefits of exercise for diabetics is the GLUT4 transporter, a protein essential for glucose uptake into cells. Found in adipose tissue and skeletal muscle, GLUT4 facilitates the entry of glucose from the bloodstream into the cells, a process crucial for maintaining blood sugar levels within a healthy range.

In diabetes, especially Type 2, GLUT4 transporter efficiency is often compromised, leading to elevated blood glucose levels. Regular exercise boosts the number and functionality of GLUT4 transporters, thereby enhancing insulin sensitivity and facilitating more effective glucose uptake. This mechanism underlies one of the key ways through which physical activity aids in controlling diabetes, making it a cornerstone of diabetes management strategy.

Enhancing Insulin Sensitivity and the Anabolic Power of Insulin

Exercise not only improves glucose uptake through the GLUT4 transporter but also enhances overall insulin sensitivity, reducing the body's need for insulin to manage blood sugar levels. Moreover, insulin's role extends beyond glucose regulation; it is a potent anabolic hormone, surpassing even testosterone in stimulating muscle growth. Insulin facilitates muscle cells' uptake of amino acids, promoting protein synthesis and muscle growth, which is crucial for maintaining muscle mass and strength, especially in individuals with diabetes.

The Multifaceted Benefits of Exercise for Diabetics

Regular physical activity offers a myriad of benefits for those managing diabetes, including:

Weight Management: Aids in achieving and maintaining a healthy weight, crucial for Type 2 diabetes management.
Improved Cardiovascular Health: Reduces the risk of heart disease, a common complication of diabetes.
Enhanced Mental Well-being: Exercise is known to improve mood and reduce stress, contributing to overall well-being.

Incorporating Exercise into Diabetes Management

Given the significant benefits, incorporating regular exercise into the routine is essential for individuals with diabetes. Whether it's aerobic activities like walking or cycling, resistance training to build muscle, or flexibility exercises such as yoga, the key is consistency and finding activities that are enjoyable and sustainable.

Chapter 13 underscores the importance of exercise in managing diabetes, spotlighting the GLUT4 transporter's role and insulin's anabolic properties. By embracing regular physical activity, individuals with diabetes can markedly improve their insulin sensitivity, manage their blood glucose levels more effectively, and enjoy a higher quality of life. Exercise, therefore, is not merely a complementary therapy but a critical component of diabetes care.

14

Exercise Bio-Hacks, Tools, and Equipment for a Better Workout Experience

I n the pursuit of optimal fitness, leveraging bio-hacks and integrating the right tools and equipment can significantly enhance your workout efficiency and experience. This chapter explores innovative bio-hacks, alongside cutting-edge tools and equipment, designed to elevate your fitness journey, streamline your workouts, and maximize your results.

Bio-Hacks for Enhanced Fitness:

Bio-hacking refers to strategic interventions that can improve physical and mental performance. Here are some effective bio-hacks to incorporate into your fitness routine:

1. High-Intensity Interval Training (HIIT): Maximizes cardiovascular and metabolic benefits in minimal time by alternating short bursts of intense exercise with periods of rest.
2. Cold Exposure: Taking cold showers or ice baths post-workout can

reduce muscle soreness and inflammation, accelerating recovery.

3. Breath Control Techniques: Incorporating breathing exercises, such as those derived from yoga, can improve oxygen efficiency, enhance endurance, and reduce stress levels.

4. Circadian Rhythm Optimization: Aligning your workout times with your body's natural circadian rhythms can improve performance and recovery. Morning workouts, for example, can help kickstart your metabolism.

5. Nutrient Timing: Consuming protein and carbohydrates within a 30-minute window after your workout can significantly enhance muscle recovery and growth.

Tools and Equipment for an Efficient Workout

The right tools and equipment can transform your workout from mundane to extraordinary, providing both motivation and improved outcomes.

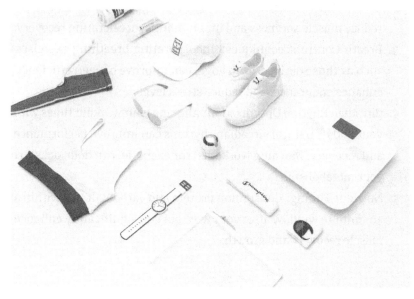

Exercise Equipment

1. Wearable Fitness Trackers: Devices like smartwatches and fitness bands track your heart rate, steps, calories burned, and sleep patterns, offering valuable insights into your performance and recovery needs.
2. Resistance Bands: Versatile and portable, resistance bands provide adjustable resistance for strength training and flexibility exercises, making them ideal for home workouts and travel.
3. Foam Rollers and Massage Guns: These recovery tools facilitate self-myofascial release, easing muscle tightness, enhancing blood flow, and reducing recovery time.
4. Adjustable Dumbbells: Space-efficient and cost-effective, adjustable dumbbells allow for a wide range of weights in one compact design, accommodating various strength levels and exercises.
5. Virtual Fitness Apps and Platforms: Digital fitness platforms offer

personalized workout plans, virtual classes, and progress tracking, providing a customizable and interactive workout experience.

6. Stability Balls and Balance Trainers: Equipment like stability balls and balance trainers challenge your core strength and stability, enhancing balance and functional fitness.

Incorporating Bio-Hacks and Tools into Your Routine

To effectively integrate these bio-hacks and tools into your fitness journey, start by identifying your specific goals and challenges. Experiment with one or two bio-hacks at a time to assess their impact on your performance and recovery. Similarly, choose tools and equipment that align with your fitness objectives, space availability, and budget.

Remember, the essence of bio-hacking and utilizing workout tools is to work smarter, not harder. By adopting these strategies and incorporating the right equipment, you can achieve greater efficiency in your workouts, enhance your overall fitness experience, and accelerate your journey towards your health and wellness goals.

15

The Importance of Body Impedance Testing

I n the realm of fitness and health optimization, understanding the intricacies of your body's composition is crucial. Body Impedance Testing (BIT), also known as Bioelectrical Impedance Analysis (BIA), stands as a pivotal tool in this understanding, offering a comprehensive glimpse into the body's internal landscape. This chapter delves into the importance of BIT, outlining its functionality and the various areas of measurement it provides, such as body fat percentage and Basal Metabolic Rate (BMR), among others.

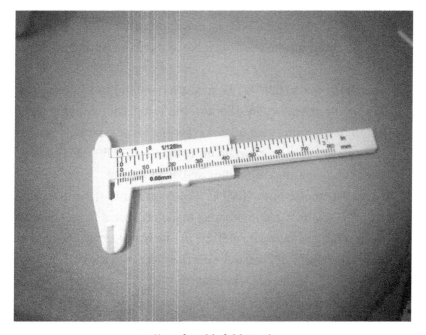

Caliper for Skinfold Testing

What is Body Impedance Testing?

BIT is a non-invasive method used to measure the composition of the body, including fat, muscle mass, and hydration levels. It operates on the principle that different body tissues conduct electrical currents to varying degrees. By passing a small, harmless electrical current through the body, BIT measures the impedance or resistance to the current flow, which is then used to calculate various body composition metrics.

Key Areas of Measurement

1. **Body Fat Percentage**: One of the most sought-after metrics, body fat percentage is crucial for assessing health and fitness levels. Unlike weight or Body Mass Index (BMI), which do not distinguish

between fat and muscle, body fat percentage offers a clearer picture of body composition, enabling more tailored fitness and nutrition strategies.

2. **Lean Body Mass (LBM)**: This measurement indicates the weight of your muscles, organs, bones, and water content, excluding fat. Understanding your LBM is essential for evaluating strength and determining appropriate nutritional and training regimens, particularly for muscle building and maintenance.

3. **Basal Metabolic Rate (BMR)**: BMR represents the number of calories your body requires at rest to maintain vital functions such as breathing, circulation, and cell production. Knowledge of your BMR is invaluable for creating effective diet plans, whether the goal is weight loss, gain, or maintenance.

4. **Total Body Water (TBW)**: TBW measurement helps assess hydration levels, crucial for overall health and performance. Proper hydration is essential for digestion, joint lubrication, and nutrient transportation.

5. **Visceral Fat Rating**: This metric quantifies the fat surrounding vital organs. High levels of visceral fat are associated with increased risks of metabolic syndromes, heart disease, and type 2 diabetes, making this measurement vital for health risk assessments.

6. **Bone Mass**: While BIT is not a direct measure of bone density, some devices estimate bone mass based on overall body composition. This information can be useful for monitoring bone health over time, especially in populations at risk of osteoporosis.

The Benefits of Regular BIT Assessments

Regular BIT assessments provide a wealth of benefits, including:

Personalized Health and Fitness Plans: By understanding your body's composition, you can tailor your fitness and nutrition plans to your specific needs, optimizing results.

Tracking Progress: BIT allows for precise tracking of changes in fat mass, muscle mass, and hydration over time, offering tangible evidence of your fitness journey's progress.

Health Risk Assessment: Measurements like visceral fat provide insights into potential health risks, enabling preventative strategies against chronic diseases.

Incorporating BIT into Your Health and Fitness Regimen

Incorporating BIT into your health and fitness regimen is straightforward with the availability of professional testing at health clubs, medical facilities, and even home-use scales and handheld devices. For accuracy, it's recommended to follow standardized conditions for testing, such as testing at the same time of day and under similar hydration and food intake conditions.

Body Impedance Testing serves as an invaluable tool in the modern fitness and health landscape. By offering a detailed analysis of body composition, BIT empowers individuals to make informed decisions about their health and fitness strategies, paving the way for more personalized and effective approaches to achieving and maintaining optimal well-being.

16

Rucking is the New Hiking

For years, I have been an advocate for a fitness activity that combines the simplicity of walking with the added challenge of weight-bearing exercise: rucking. This chapter will delve into the essence of rucking, a practice that redefines traditional hiking by introducing the element of carrying weight, making it an efficient, full-body workout. We'll explore how to incorporate rucking into your routine, even on a budget, the extensive benefits it offers, and how a weighted vest can transform gym workouts.

What is Rucking?

Rucking is essentially walking or hiking while carrying additional weight, typically in a backpack. Originating from military training, where soldiers carry heavy packs across varied terrains, rucking has gained popularity among civilians as a straightforward yet effective fitness regimen. Unlike traditional hiking, the added weight in rucking increases the exercise intensity, engaging more muscle groups, and burning more calories.

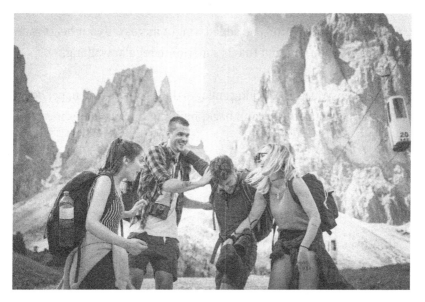

Rucking/Hiking with Friends.

Incorporating Household Items for Rucking

Not everyone has access to specialized equipment like weighted vests or ruck plates, but that shouldn't deter you from exploring rucking. Household items such as water bottles, sandbags, or even books can serve as weights. Place these items in a sturdy backpack, ensuring the weight is evenly distributed to avoid strain on your back. Start with a weight you're comfortable with, ideally 10% of your body weight, and gradually increase as your endurance and strength improve.

The Benefits of Rucking

Rucking offers a myriad of benefits, making it a comprehensive workout choice for individuals of all fitness levels:

1. Cardiovascular Health: The added weight increases your heart rate, providing a cardio workout that is superior to regular walking.

2. Strengthens Muscles: Rucking engages the legs, core, and upper body, particularly the shoulders and back, building muscle endurance and strength.

3. Burns Calories: The combination of cardio and strength training ensures high calorie burn, aiding in weight management and fat loss.

4. Improves Posture: Carrying weight requires you to maintain good posture, strengthening the back and shoulder muscles responsible for alignment.

5. Mental Health: Like hiking, rucking offers mental health benefits through outdoor exercise, reducing stress, and enhancing mood.

6. Accessibility and Versatility: Rucking can be done anywhere, from city streets to hiking trails, making it a versatile workout that fits various lifestyles and preferences.

Using a Weighted Vest in the Gym

Beyond rucking, a weighted vest can be a valuable tool in the gym, adding intensity to a wide range of exercises. Here's how to incorporate it:

Bodyweight Exercises: Perform squats, push-ups, lunges, and pull-ups with a weighted vest to increase resistance and challenge your muscles.

Cardio Workouts: Wearing a vest while on a treadmill, stair climber, or during high-intensity interval training (HIIT) significantly boosts cardio intensity and calorie burn.

Core Training: Exercises like planks or mountain climbers with added weight enhance core engagement and strength.

Rucking, with its simplicity and effectiveness, stands as a testament to the idea that fitness doesn't need to be complicated or expensive. Whether you're traversing a mountain trail with a weighted pack or integrating a weighted vest into your gym routine, the principle remains the same: adding weight transforms ordinary activities into profound workouts. As we embrace rucking as the new hiking, we unlock a pathway to enhanced physical fitness, mental clarity, and overall well-being, proving that sometimes, the best way forward is to carry a little weight on our shoulders.

17

Glycolysis vs. Lypolysis: Understanding Energy Pathways

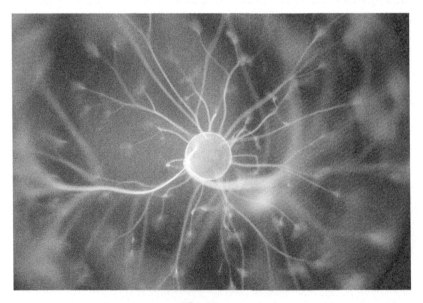

Bio-Energy

In the quest for fitness and optimal health, understanding the body's energy systems is crucial. Two key processes at the heart of these systems are glycolysis and lipolysis. Both are essential for energy production but operate in distinct ways and under different conditions. This chapter will delve into the differences between these processes, explore the body's energy pathways, and elucidate the mechanisms behind burning carbohydrates versus fat for energy.

Glycolysis: The Carbohydrate Energy Pathway

Glycolysis is the process by which glucose, a simple sugar derived from carbohydrates, is broken down in the body's cells to produce energy. It is the initial step in the broader metabolic pathway of cellular respiration, which generates ATP (adenosine triphosphate), the energy currency of the cell. Glycolysis occurs in the cytoplasm of cells and does not require oxygen, making it an anaerobic process.

During glycolysis, one molecule of glucose is converted into two molecules of pyruvate. This conversion results in a net gain of two ATP molecules, which are used by the body for short, high-intensity activities lasting from a few seconds to about two minutes. The speed at which ATP can be produced makes glycolysis highly efficient for immediate energy needs.

Lipolysis: The Fat Energy Pathway

In contrast, lipolysis is the process of breaking down triglycerides (the main form of body fat) into glycerol and free fatty acids, which can then be used for energy. Lipolysis primarily occurs in adipose (fat) tissue and is influenced by hormonal signals in response to energy demand.

The free fatty acids released during lipolysis can enter the mitochondria of cells, where they undergo beta-oxidation to produce acetyl-CoA. Acetyl-CoA then enters the citric acid cycle (Krebs cycle), followed by the electron transport chain, where a significant amount of ATP is generated. Unlike glycolysis, lipolysis and subsequent fat oxidation require oxygen, making it an aerobic process.

Because the breakdown of fat for energy is slower and more complex than the breakdown of glucose, lipolysis is primarily utilized during prolonged, low to moderate intensity activities. It is highly efficient for sustained energy production over longer periods.

Energy Pathways: Aerobic vs. Anaerobic

The body switches between aerobic and anaerobic energy pathways based on oxygen availability and the intensity of physical activity. Glycolysis provides quick energy in anaerobic conditions, such as during a sprint or heavy lifting, when the demand for ATP exceeds the oxygen available for fat oxidation. Conversely, during aerobic activities like long-distance running or cycling, the body relies more on lipolysis and fat oxidation, which are more oxygen-dependent but produce ATP more sustainably.

Burning Carbohydrates vs. Burning Fat for Energy

The choice between burning carbohydrates (glycolysis) and burning fat (lipolysis) is influenced by several factors, including exercise intensity, duration, and the individual's metabolic state. Glycolysis is favored for quick, intense energy bursts, relying on glucose stores in the muscles and liver. In contrast, lipolysis is favored during prolonged, steady-state exercise, tapping into the body's abundant fat stores for a more sustained energy release.

Understanding the differences between glycolysis and lipolysis, and how the body selects and utilizes these energy pathways, is fundamental for optimizing workout strategies, dietary choices, and overall energy management. By aligning your fitness and nutrition plans with these metabolic processes, you can enhance your performance, improve endurance, and better achieve your health and fitness goals.

18

Conclusion

As we close this chapter, and not just of the book but of our journey together it's time to reflect on the ground we've covered and look forward to the path that lies ahead. The essence of this guide has been to equip you with the knowledge, inspiration, and tools necessary to embrace active aging, to show that maintaining fitness and well-being in your 40's, 50's, and 60's is not just a possibility but a profound opportunity.

Key Takeaways

Holistic Fitness is Key: We've explored the importance of combining strength training, cardiovascular exercises, flexibility, and mobility work to create a balanced fitness regimen that supports overall health and well-being.

Adaptability and Personalization: Your fitness journey is uniquely yours. Tailoring your workout routine to fit your individual needs, preferences, and challenges is crucial for sustainable success.

Prevention and Recovery: Understanding the importance of injury prevention, recognizing when to seek professional advice, and adopting effective recovery practices ensure that you can enjoy a lifetime of activity.

Mindset Matters: Perhaps the most critical lesson is the power of a positive mindset. Embracing challenges, celebrating progress, and staying motivated are essential components of a fulfilling fitness journey.

Embracing and Prioritizing Your Fitness and Well-Being

The journey of active aging is not just about adding years to your life but life to your years. It's about enhancing your quality of life, enabling you to pursue your passions, enjoy your achievements, and share memorable moments with loved ones. Prioritizing your fitness and well-being is the greatest gift you can give yourself and those around you.

A Final Word of Encouragement

If there's one message to carry with you, let it be this: It's never too late to start, but it's always too early to give up. Whether you're taking your first steps towards a more active lifestyle or seeking to reach new heights in your fitness journey, believe in your ability to achieve your goals. The path may not always be easy, but the rewards are strength, vitality, and a deeper appreciation for your body's capabilities are immeasurable.

Remember, aging is an inevitable part of life, but how we age is something we can influence. Embrace the opportunity to age actively, with grace, strength, and an indomitable spirit. Your fitness journey in your 40's, 50's, and 60's is not just about extending your years but enriching them, transforming this chapter of your life into one of the most rewarding yet.

As you turn the page from this book to the next chapter of your fitness journey, go forth with confidence, determination, and a heart full of adventure. The best is yet to come...

References

Haff, G. G. (2016). Essentials of Strength Training and Conditioning, 4th Edition. *Medicine and Science in Sports and Exercise*, 48(10), 2073. https://doi.org/10.1249/mss.0000000000001081

Jessen, N., & Goodyear, L. J. (2005). GLUT4 and its role in diabetes and metabolism. Trends in Endocrinology and Metabolism, 16(6), 259-266. https://doi:10.1016/j.tem.2005.06.004

U.S. Department of Health and Human Services and U.S. Department of Agriculture. (2020). Dietary Guidelines for Americans. Retrieved from https://www.dietaryguidelines.gov/sites/default/files/2020-12/ Dietary_Guidelines_for_Americans_2020-2025.pdf

Houtkooper, L. B., Lohman, T. G., Going, S. B., Howell, W. H., & Roche, A. F. (1996). Bioelectrical impedance estimation of fat-free body mass in children and youth: a cross-validation study. Journal of Applied Physiology, 80(3), 847-852

Xu, K., Hong, Y., & Li, X. (2019). Lipolysis and glycolysis: key metabolic pathways involved in the regulation of adipose tissue metabolism and insulin sensitivity. Adipocyte, 8(1), 275-285. https://doi:10.1080/21623 945.2019.1654281

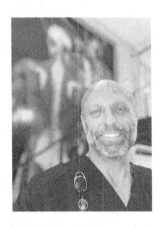

About the Author

The journey of our author is a profound testament to human resilience, a real-life saga that exemplifies the saying, "What Doesn't Kill You, Makes You Stronger." This phrase is not merely a motivational quote for him but a lived reality, a guiding light through the darkest tunnels of life-threatening medical challenges and towards the dawn of personal reinvention and triumph.

Christopher's odyssey into the abyss began innocuously in 2008 with a diagnosis of a benign cyst. What was anticipated to be a straightforward outpatient procedure spiraled into an unforeseen medical catastrophe. Complications arose when an infection, a silent predator, invaded the surgical site, ravaging his right hip, pelvis, and femur, and thrusting his body into a lethal dance with sepsis. The dire situation necessitated a medically induced coma, an intervention that marked the commencement of a grueling two-year battle for mere survival. Upon awakening, encumbered by a labyrinth of wires and tubes, he found himself on the precipice of a long, arduous journey back to health. Confined to home traction without the structural integrity of bones in his right leg, his resilience was put to the ultimate test. It was the unparalleled skill and dedication of the medical teams at U.S.C.'s Keck School of Medicine and Rancho Los Amigos Hospital that engineered his "reconstruction." Yet, the victory of relearning to walk belied the enduring battles ahead.

The aftermath of his medical ordeal left an indelible mark on his physical form and quality of life. He emerged with severe disabilities and a daily companion of chronic pain, mitigated only by the continuous hum of a neuro-stimulator implant woven into his spinal cord. The very medications that had been his lifeline through this storm wreaked havoc on his body, annihilating his pancreas and precipitating diabetes. In 2013, he faced another formidable foe: Endocrine Pancreatic Insufficiency, a condition that rendered his pancreas incapable of producing essential enzymes, thus imperiling his life once more. The ensuing battle required him to rely on IV feeding for sustenance, a testament to his unyielding spirit.

Yet, amidst the relentless onslaught of health crises, a pivotal moment of clarity emerged in January 2015. With unwavering determination, he resolved to take the reins of his health, venturing into a disciplined regime of exercise and nutritional overhaul. This decision, however, was not without its sacrifices. The pursuit of education and a semblance of normalcy came at a steep price, including the loss of federal disability benefits and the sale of his car to fund medications and school expenses.

The author's journey is a vivid illustration of resilience, determination, and an unwavering commitment to health and fitness. Not only has he navigated through a labyrinth of personal health crises with remarkable fortitude, but he has also transformed these experiences into a catalyst for profound personal and professional growth. His narrative extends beyond his battles with health issues, unfolding into a story of triumph and relentless pursuit of knowledge.

After overcoming significant medical hurdles, Christopher turned adversity into opportunity by deciding to go back to college. His passion for understanding the human body and its potential for recovery and optimization led him to immerse himself in the study of Kinesiology. Through dedication and hard work, he obtained multiple degrees in this field, laying a solid foundation for his career in health and fitness.

But Christopher didn't stop there. His quest for knowledge led him to acquire certifications in the medical field, further broadening his expertise and ability to help others. His certifications have enabled him to blend scientific knowledge with practical application, making a tangible difference in people's lives.

Currently, Christopher excels as a personal trainer, nutritionist, physiotherapist, massage, and lymphatic therapist. In these roles, he combines his in-depth understanding of human physiology with a personalized approach to help his clients achieve their health and fitness goals. His work is not just about physical transformation; it's about empowering individuals to reclaim their health and vitality, much like he did.

Christopher is also on an ambitious path to further his education. He is working towards obtaining his Bachelor's degree in Exercise Science, a field that encompasses the breadth of knowledge he is passionate about. Additionally, he is in the process of receiving his strength and conditioning certification, a testament to his commitment to excellence and his desire to provide the highest level of service to his clients.

Through his academic achievements, professional certifications, and personal journey back to health, Christopher embodies the principles he teaches. His life is a powerful narrative of overcoming adversity through resilience, education, and the transformative power of fitness. As an author, personal trainer, nutritionist, physio, massage, and lymphatic therapist, he stands as a beacon of hope and a source of inspiration for anyone looking to overcome their own challenges and achieve optimal health and wellness.

You can connect with me on:

🌐 https://www.zeebodyworkandlymphaticmedicine.com

📘 https://www.facebook.com/profile.php?id=61556377641370

🔗 http://linkedin.com/in/christopher-zanderholm-760076292

🔗 https://www.tiktok.com/@zeeathletics?_t=8lyPTxqW3ER&_r=1

🔗 https://www.zeeathleticsanddietetics.com

🔗 https://www.instagram.com/swedefromthemeade75

Made in United States
Orlando, FL
20 December 2024

56239368R00065